NATURAL WEIGHT LOSS

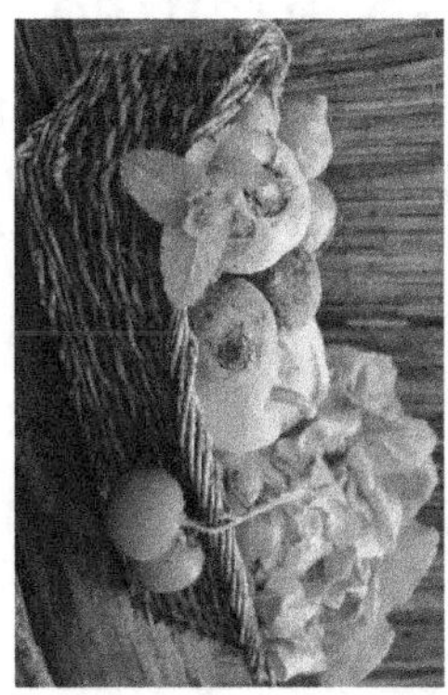

"Harmony in Health: Embracing Natural Paths to Weight Wellness"

Temmy Brown

COPYRIGHT

(2024) Copyright © Temmy Brown

All rights reserved.Except for limited nonprofit uses permitted by copyright law and brief quotes in critical reviews, no portion of this publication may be copied, shared, or transmitted in any form without the publisher's prior written authorization. Photocopying, recording, and other mechanical or electronic techniques are prohibited.

Table Of Content 5

Introduction: **10**

CHAPTER ONE **12**

A. Embracing Natural Approaches: 12

B. Importance of Sustainable Weight Loss: 13

CHAPTER TWO **15**

Whole Foods and Nutrient-Rich Diets 15

A. Plant-Based Eating: 15

B. Incorporating Fruits and Vegetables: 16

C. Lean Proteins and Healthy Fats: 17

CHAPTER THREE **19**

Hydration 19

A. Importance of Water for Weight Loss: 19

B. Herbal Infusion and Tea: 21

C. Limiting Sugary Beverages: 22

CHAPTER FOUR **24**

Mindful Eating 24

A.What is mindful eating? 24

B. Mindful Meal Practices: 26

C. Avoiding Emotional Eating: 27

CHAPTER FIVE **28**

Physical Activity in Nature 28

A. Outdoor Exercises: 28

B. Hiking, Walking, and Running: 29

C. Connecting with Nature for Mental Health: 30

CHAPTER SIX **32**

Herbal Supplements and Natural Remedies 32
    A. Green Tea and Weight Loss: 32
    B. Natural Metabolism Boosters: 33
    C. Considerations and Caution: 34
CHAPTER SEVEN **36**
Stress Management 36
    A. Impact of Stress on Weight: 36
    B. Relaxation Techniques: 37
    C. Incorporating Mind-Body Practices: 37
CHAPTER EIGHT **39**
Adequate Sleep 39
    A. Sleep and Metabolism: 39
    B. Establishing Healthy Sleep Patterns: 40
    C. Creating a Restful Sleep Environment: 40
CHAPTER NINE **42**
Gut Health 42
    A. Probiotics and Prebiotics: 42
    B. Fermented Foods: 43
    C. Gut-Brain Connection: 44
CHAPTER TEN **45**
Portion Control 45
    A. Recognizing Serving Sizes: 45
    B. Using Smaller Plates: 46
    C. Mindful Portioning Techniques: 46
CHAPTER ELEVEN **47**
Natural Weight Loss Herbs and Spices 48
    A. Thermogenic Herbs: 48
    B. Appetite-Suppressing Spices: 49

C. Integrating Flavorful Options: 49

CHAPTER TWELVE   **50**

Community and Social Support   51

A. Importance of a Support System: 51

B. Group Activities and Accountability: 51

C. Sharing Experiences and Success Stories: 53

CHAPTER THIRTEEN   **54**

Sustainable Lifestyle Changes   54

A. Gradual Progress Over Quick Fixes: 54

B. Creating Lasting Habits: 55

C. Balancing Enjoyment and Health: 56

Conclusion   **57**

A. Emphasizing Holistic and Natural Approaches: 57

B. Encouragement for a Healthier Lifestyle: 58

Introduction:

In the quest for a healthier and more balanced life, the journey toward natural weight loss stands as a pivotal gateway to overall well-being. This introduction sets the stage for exploring sustainable approaches, emphasizing the interconnectedness of nutrition, physical activity, mindfulness, and lifestyle choices. As we delve into the realms of whole foods, mindful eating, and the nurturing of our body's innate capacities, this guide aims to inspire a transformative shift toward lasting health and vitality. Join us on this empowering exploration of natural weight loss, where the focus is not just on shedding pounds but on cultivating

7

a harmonious and sustainable
relationship with our bodies.

CHAPTER ONE

A. Embracing Natural Approaches:

Embarking on a journey of natural weight loss involves a fundamental shift in perspective towards the nourishment and care of our bodies. In this section, we delve into the principles of whole foods and nutrient-rich diets, exploring the benefits of embracing plant-based eating, incorporating an abundance of fruits and vegetables, and understanding the importance of lean proteins and healthy fats. By adopting a holistic approach rooted in the goodness of nature, we lay the foundation for a sustainable and nourishing transformation, promoting not only weight loss but overall well-being.

B. Importance of Sustainable Weight Loss:

Within the realm of natural weight loss, sustainability emerges as a guiding principle. This section underscores the significance of adopting practices that go beyond quick fixes, crash diets, and temporary solutions. We delve into the long-term implications of sustainable weight loss, emphasizing the importance of making lifestyle changes that can be maintained over time. By acknowledging the interconnectedness of nutrition, physical activity, and mental well-being, we pave the way for a journey that not only achieves weight loss goals but cultivates enduring health and balance. Explore the transformative power of sustainable choices as we navigate the path to a healthier, more fulfilling life.

CHAPTER TWO

Whole Foods and Nutrient-Rich Diets

A. Plant-Based Eating:

In the pursuit of natural weight loss, adopting a plant-based eating approach emerges as a cornerstone. This involves prioritizing whole, plant-derived foods such as fruits, vegetables, legumes, nuts, and seeds. Plant-based diets are rich in fiber, vitamins, and minerals, offering a myriad of health benefits. The emphasis on plant-based eating is not only conducive to weight loss but also contributes to improved digestion, increased energy levels, and a reduced risk of chronic diseases. This section delves into the principles of plant-based nutrition, providing insights into crafting a well-balanced and satisfying diet centered around nature's bountiful offerings.

B. Incorporating Fruits and Vegetables:

Fruits and vegetables play a pivotal role in a nutrient-rich diet that supports natural weight loss. This subsection explores the diverse array of vitamins, minerals, and antioxidants found in these colorful, plant-based foods. From leafy greens packed with essential nutrients to vibrant berries known for their antioxidant properties, we delve into the nutritional benefits of incorporating a variety of fruits and vegetables into daily meals. Practical tips on meal planning, creative recipes, and strategies to maximize nutritional intake form the foundation of this exploration into the vibrant world of plant-centric nutrition.

C. Lean Proteins and Healthy Fats:

Balancing macronutrients is key to sustaining a healthy and effective weight loss journey. This section focuses on the importance of incorporating lean proteins and healthy fats into the diet. Lean proteins, sourced from poultry, fish, legumes, and plant-based sources, provide essential amino acids crucial for muscle maintenance and satiety. Simultaneously, healthy fats derived from avocados, nuts, seeds, and olive oil contribute to overall well-being, supporting cognitive function and aiding in the absorption of fat-soluble vitamins. By understanding the role of these macronutrients, individuals can create a satisfying and nutritionally dense eating plan that fosters natural weight loss while promoting overall health.

CHAPTER THREE

Hydration

A. Importance of Water for Weight Loss:

Water, often overlooked in weight loss discussions, plays a pivotal role in supporting natural and sustainable weight loss. This subsection delves into the significance of staying adequately hydrated for optimal metabolic function and appetite regulation. Water intake helps in the digestion and absorption of nutrients, aids in the elimination of waste products, and can contribute to a feeling of fullness, reducing the likelihood of overeating. By understanding the crucial role of water in the body's processes, individuals

can harness its benefits as a
fundamental aspect of their weight
loss journey.

water drinking can help burn calories
and reduce hunger cravings.
Replacement of sugary drinks with
water can also lower caloric and sugar
intake. But water drinking alone is not
enough for major weight loss.

When drinking cold water, your body
uses extra calories to warm the water
up to body temperature.

B. Herbal Infusion and Tea:
Herbal drinks play a vital role in losing
weight by offering low-calorie,
hydrating alternatives to sugary
beverages. Herbal infusions, such as

ginger or peppermint tea, can aid digestion and reduce cravings.

Beyond plain water, herbal teas and infusions present a flavorful and healthful approach to hydration. This section explores the diverse array of herbal teas and infusions that not only contribute to hydration but also offer additional health benefits. From metabolism-boosting teas to those known for their calming effects, herbal infusions can be integrated into a weight loss plan to enhance overall well-being. Practical tips on brewing and incorporating these beverages into daily routines add a refreshing dimension to the hydration aspect of natural weight loss.

C. Limiting Sugary Beverages:

An essential component of a holistic approach to hydration and weight loss involves being mindful of beverage choices. This subsection sheds light on the detrimental impact of sugary beverages on weight management and overall health. By understanding the hidden calories and potential metabolic disruptions caused by excessive sugar intake, individuals can make informed choices to limit or eliminate sugary drinks from their diet. Practical strategies for reducing reliance on sugary beverages and alternatives that support hydration without compromising health goals are explored to empower individuals in their journey towards natural weight loss.

Artificial drinks are chemical additives that are sweeter than sugar but add very little energy to the diet and therefore do not contribute directly to weight gain. However, artificial drinks still maintain the 'habit' of drinking sweet drinks and there is some evidence that consumption of all soft drinks, both diet and sugar–sweetened, may lead to decreased bone density as people may drink less milk.

CHAPTER FOUR

Mindful Eating

A. What is mindful eating?

Mindful eating is a practice that involves paying full attention to the experience of eating, including the sensations, flavors, and emotions associated with each bite. It encourages being present in the moment, savoring food, and recognizing hunger and fullness cues. This approach can help foster a healthier relationship with food and promote better overall well-being. Mindfulness is a form of meditation that helps you recognize and cope with

your emotions and physical sensations.
Mindful eating is about developing awareness of your experiences, physical cues, and feelings about food.
A. Understanding Hunger and Fullness:

Mindful eating forms a foundational element of natural weight loss, focusing on the awareness of hunger and fullness signals. This subsection delves into the importance of reconnecting with the body's natural cues for hunger and fullness. By tuning into sensations of physical hunger, individuals can make informed and intentional choices about when and how much to eat. The practice of mindful eating encourages a deeper appreciation for the nourishment derived from food, fostering a healthier relationship with eating and promoting sustainable weight loss.

B. Mindful Meal Practices:

This section explores practical strategies for incorporating mindful practices into meals. From savoring the flavors and textures of food to paying attention to portion sizes, mindful meal practices aim to enhance the overall eating experience. Techniques such as slowing down the pace of eating, eliminating distractions, and engaging the senses contribute to a heightened awareness of the act of consuming food. By cultivating mindfulness during meals, individuals can derive greater satisfaction from their food, leading to a more mindful and intentional approach to nourishment that supports natural weight loss.

C. Avoiding Emotional Eating:

Emotional eating can be a significant obstacle on the path to natural weight loss. This subsection addresses the connection between emotions and eating habits, offering insights into identifying emotional triggers and developing alternative coping mechanisms. Strategies for recognizing and addressing emotional hunger versus physical hunger are explored, empowering individuals to make conscious choices about their food intake. By fostering a greater understanding of the emotional aspects of eating, individuals can cultivate resilience and develop

23

healthier responses to emotional triggers, contributing to a more balanced and mindful approach to nourishment.

CHAPTER FIVE

Physical Activity in Nature

A. Outdoor Exercises:

Embracing the great outdoors becomes a dynamic catalyst for natural weight loss through a diverse range of outdoor exercises. This section explores the advantages of incorporating activities like cycling, calisthenics, or group workouts in natural settings. By leveraging the varied terrain and fresh air, outdoor exercises not only enhance physical fitness but also provide an invigorating and inspiring backdrop for the journey towards a healthier, more active lifestyle. Practical tips on adapting workouts to outdoor environments and maximizing the benefits of nature are woven into this exploration of fitness beyond the confines of a gym.

B. Hiking, Walking, and Running:

The simplicity and accessibility of hiking, walking, and running make them integral components of a nature-infused fitness routine. This subsection delves into the unique advantages of these activities, from the cardiovascular benefits of brisk walking to the endurance-building aspects of trail running. Practical advice on gear, pacing, and gradually increasing intensity encourages individuals to harness the power of these natural movements. Whether strolling through scenic trails or pushing personal limits in a jog, the focus is on making these activities not just exercises but enjoyable pursuits that contribute to natural weight loss.

C. Connecting with Nature for Mental Health:

Beyond the physical exertion, connecting with nature during physical activity proves to be a potent tonic for mental well-being. This segment explores the symbiotic relationship between exercise and nature, elucidating how the outdoor environment enhances mental health. From reducing stress to boosting mood and fostering a sense of tranquility, the mental health benefits of nature-infused physical activity are highlighted. By recognizing the intertwined harmony between physical exertion and the natural world, individuals can embark on a holistic approach to weight loss that nurtures both body and mind.

CHAPTER SIX

Herbal Supplements and Natural Remedies

A. Green Tea and Weight Loss:

Green tea stands out as a popular herbal supplement renowned for its potential role in supporting natural weight loss. This section explores the mechanisms behind green tea's impact on metabolism and fat burning. Rich in antioxidants, particularly catechins, green tea is believed to enhance calorie expenditure and contribute to weight management. Practical tips on incorporating green tea into a daily routine and understanding its potential benefits form the foundation of this exploration into one of nature's well-regarded herbal remedies for weight loss.

B. Natural Metabolism Boosters:

This subsection delves into a variety of natural metabolism boosters that may aid in the quest for weight loss. From spices like cayenne pepper to foods like ginger and certain herbal supplements, the focus is on understanding how these natural elements may enhance metabolic function. Practical considerations such as proper dosage, potential side effects, and incorporating these boosters into a balanced diet are discussed. By exploring these natural allies, individuals can make informed choices to support their metabolism in a way that aligns with their overall health goals.

C. Considerations and Caution:

While herbal supplements and natural remedies offer potential benefits, it's crucial to approach them with consideration and caution. This section provides guidance on factors to consider before incorporating herbal supplements, including individual health conditions, potential interactions with medications, and consulting healthcare professionals. The importance of obtaining herbal products from reputable sources and being mindful of dosage is emphasized. By promoting informed decision-making and acknowledging potential risks, this section aims to empower individuals to navigate the realm of herbal supplements responsibly as part of their natural weight loss journey.

CHAPTER SEVEN

Stress Management

A. Impact of Stress on Weight:

This section delves into the intricate relationship between stress and weight, highlighting how chronic stress can disrupt hormonal balance and contribute to weight gain. By understanding the physiological mechanisms at play, individuals can appreciate the importance of stress management in supporting natural weight loss. Insightful information on cortisol, the stress hormone, and its implications for metabolism provides a foundation for adopting effective stress reduction strategies.

B. Relaxation Techniques:

To Explore a range of relaxation techniques, this subsection offers practical approaches to alleviate stress and its potential impact on weight. Techniques such as deep breathing, progressive muscle relaxation, and guided imagery are discussed for their effectiveness in promoting relaxation and reducing stress levels. Incorporating these techniques into daily routines empowers individuals to build resilience against stressors, fostering a balanced mental and emotional state conducive to natural weight loss.

C. Incorporating Mind-Body Practices:

Mind-body practices, including yoga, tai chi, and meditation, offer holistic approaches to stress management and weight loss. This part explores the benefits of integrating these practices into a wellness routine. By emphasizing the mind-body connection, individuals can enhance self-awareness, reduce stress-related eating, and cultivate a mindful approach to their overall well-being. Practical tips on starting and sustaining mind-body practices contribute to a comprehensive strategy for stress management on the journey to natural weight loss.

CHAPTER EIGHT

Adequate Sleep

A. Sleep and Metabolism:

This section delves into the intricate relationship between sleep and metabolism, exploring how inadequate sleep can impact hormonal regulation and disrupt metabolic processes. The subsection highlights the importance of sufficient and quality sleep in supporting natural weight loss. By understanding the role of sleep in appetite control and energy balance, individuals gain insights into optimizing their sleep patterns to foster a healthier metabolism.

B. Establishing Healthy Sleep Patterns:

Practical guidance on establishing healthy sleep patterns forms a crucial aspect of this exploration. The section offers tips for creating a consistent sleep schedule, optimizing sleep duration, and adopting pre-sleep routines to signal the body for rest. Strategies for managing factors like screen time, caffeine intake, and evening activities contribute to the development of sustainable and health-promoting sleep habits, which are crucial for those seeking to achieve and maintain natural weight loss.

C. Creating a Restful Sleep Environment:

The impact of the sleep environment on sleep quality is underscored in this subsection. Practical considerations for creating a restful sleep environment, including optimizing room temperature, minimizing noise and light, and choosing comfortable bedding, are explored. By fostering a sleep-conducive environment, individuals can enhance the quality of their sleep, supporting the body's natural processes and contributing to overall health and successful weight management.

CHAPTER NINE

Gut Health

A. Probiotics and Prebiotics:

This section explores the dynamic world of gut health, beginning with the roles of probiotics and prebiotics. It delves into the benefits of probiotics, which are beneficial bacteria that support a healthy gut microbiome. Prebiotics, on the other hand, provide the necessary nourishment for these beneficial bacteria. Practical insights into incorporating probiotic-rich foods like yogurt and fermented vegetables, as well as prebiotic sources such as fiber-rich foods, offer a comprehensive approach to fostering gut health in the context of natural weight loss, adding a prebiotic or probiotic supplement to your diet may help improve your gut health.

B. Fermented Foods:

Fermented foods take center stage as natural contributors to a flourishing gut environment. This subsection examines the diverse array of fermented foods, including kimchi, sauerkraut, and kefir, and their potential impact on gut health. The section provides practical advice on incorporating these foods into a balanced diet, offering not only digestive benefits but also potential support for weight management through the gut microbiota's influence on metabolism. Fermented foods are great dietary sources of probiotics.

C. Gut-Brain Connection:

The intricate interplay between gut health and mental well-being is explored in this part. Understanding the gut-brain connection sheds light on how gut health influences mood, cravings, and overall mental health, which can impact eating behaviors and, subsequently, weight management. Insights into how a healthy gut contributes to a positive mindset and supports the journey of natural weight loss form the foundation of this exploration into the complex and fascinating relationship between the gut and the brain.

CHAPTER TEN

Portion Control

A. Recognizing Serving Sizes:

This section addresses the importance of recognizing appropriate serving sizes as a fundamental aspect of natural weight loss. It explores practical strategies for understanding portion sizes, such as using visual cues and learning to estimate appropriate amounts. By enhancing awareness of serving sizes, individuals can make informed choices, manage caloric intake, and foster a balanced approach to nutrition.

B. Using Smaller Plates:

The utilization of smaller plates is presented as a strategic tool for portion control. This subsection delves into the psychological impact of plate size on perceived portion sizes, exploring how using smaller plates can create an illusion of larger servings. Practical advice on implementing this technique in everyday meals is provided, offering a simple yet effective approach to managing portion sizes without sacrificing satisfaction.

C. Mindful Portioning Techniques:

Mindful portioning techniques form an integral part of this exploration into portion control. The section discusses practices such as eating slowly, savoring each bite, and paying attention to hunger and fullness cues. By cultivating mindfulness during meals, individuals can develop a deeper connection with their eating habits, making it easier to adopt portion control as a sustainable and enjoyable aspect of their natural weight loss journey.

CHAPTER ELEVEN

Natural Weight Loss Herbs and Spices

A. Thermogenic Herbs:

This section introduces the concept of thermogenic herbs—plants that may boost metabolism and contribute to natural weight loss. The exploration delves into specific herbs, such as cayenne pepper and green tea, known for their thermogenic properties. Practical insights into incorporating these herbs into daily meals and understanding their potential impact on metabolic processes offer a holistic approach to utilizing nature's thermogenic allies for weight management.

B. Appetite-Suppressing Spices:

The spotlight turns to appetite-suppressing spices in this subsection, unveiling flavorful options that may aid in controlling cravings and promoting satiety. Spices like cinnamon, ginger, and fenugreek are discussed for their potential impact on appetite regulation. Practical tips on integrating these spices into various dishes provide individuals with creative and enjoyable ways to leverage natural appetite-suppressing properties in their culinary endeavors.

C. Integrating Flavorful Options:

Balancing the pursuit of natural weight loss with flavorful and satisfying options is the focus of this part. The section explores the synergy between herbs, spices, and the enjoyment of food. By highlighting diverse and flavorful options, individuals can enhance their culinary experiences while supporting their weight loss goals. Practical suggestions for incorporating a variety of herbs and spices into meals provide a roadmap for achieving both taste and health in a harmonious manner.

CHAPTER TWELVE

Community and Social Support

A. Importance of a Support System:

This section emphasizes the pivotal role of a support system in the natural weight loss journey. It explores the psychological and motivational benefits of having a network of individuals who provide encouragement, understanding, and accountability. Insights into the significance of emotional support and shared experiences create a foundation for individuals to recognize and actively seek out a supportive community.

B. Group Activities and Accountability:

What is accountability in weight loss? Accountability is an obligation or willingness to accept responsibility for one's actions." Awareness is very important when it comes to accomplishing our goals.

Engaging in group activities and fostering accountability within a community setting forms a key aspect of this exploration. The subsection delves into the benefits of participating in group workouts, classes, or weight loss challenges. The sense of accountability that arises from shared goals and activities encourages consistency and commitment. Practical tips for incorporating group activities into one's routine contribute to the establishment of a supportive and active community.

C. Sharing Experiences and Success Stories:

The power of sharing experiences and success stories is highlighted in this part. By encouraging individuals to share their triumphs and challenges, a sense of camaraderie and inspiration is cultivated within the community. This exchange of narratives serves as a motivational tool, providing real-world examples of achievement and resilience. Practical insights into

creating platforms for sharing
experiences contribute to the
development of a positive and uplifting
community dedicated to natural
weight loss.

CHAPTER THIRTEEN

Sustainable Lifestyle Changes

A. Gradual Progress Over Quick Fixes:

This section advocates for a gradual and sustainable approach to natural weight loss, emphasizing the importance of making lasting changes over seeking quick fixes. It explores the pitfalls of rapid weight loss methods and encourages individuals to focus on making small, manageable adjustments to their lifestyle. By embracing a mindset of gradual progress, individuals can build a foundation for long-term success in achieving and maintaining a healthier weight.

B. Creating Lasting Habits:

The establishment of lasting habits is at the core of sustainable lifestyle changes. This subsection explores the science of habit formation and provides practical strategies for cultivating behaviors that contribute to natural weight loss. From setting achievable goals to incorporating new habits into daily routines, the emphasis is on creating a sustainable and supportive environment that promotes the integration of healthy behaviors into one's lifestyle.

C. Balancing Enjoyment and Health:

Maintaining a balance between enjoyment and health is a key theme in this part. The section explores the importance of finding joy in the journey and embracing foods and activities that bring satisfaction while aligning with health goals. Practical insights into mindful indulgence, occasional treats, and flexible approaches to dietary choices contribute to the creation of a balanced and sustainable lifestyle. By fostering a positive relationship with both health and enjoyment, individuals can navigate the path to natural weight loss with a sense of fulfillment and long-term well-being.

Conclusion

A. Emphasizing Holistic and Natural Approaches:

As we conclude this guide, the overarching theme underscores the significance of embracing holistic and natural approaches to weight loss. The exploration of whole foods, physical activity in nature, stress management, and the integration of herbs and spices have woven together a comprehensive tapestry of health. By emphasizing the interconnectedness of these elements, individuals are encouraged to view weight loss not as a singular pursuit but as part of a broader journey toward holistic well-being.

B. Encouragement for a Healthier Lifestyle:

The final words of this guide are dedicated to offering encouragement for embracing a healthier lifestyle. Recognizing that the pursuit of natural weight loss is not solely about shedding pounds but about fostering lasting health and vitality, individuals are empowered to embark on a journey that prioritizes well-being. The encouragement extends beyond the physical aspects to encompass mental and emotional wellness, emphasizing that a healthier lifestyle is not only attainable but a rewarding and fulfilling endeavor. May this guide catalyze positive change, inspiring individuals to embrace natural approaches and embark on a path toward a healthier and more vibrant life.

www.ingramcontent.com/pod-product-compliance
Lightning Source LLC
Chambersburg PA
CBHW071000250726
48663CB00002B/311

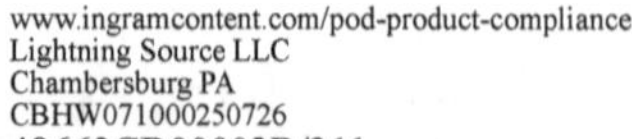